THIS BOOK BELONGS TO:

_____

_____

Copyright © 2021 by Ava Smith

All rights reserved. No part of this publication may be reproduced, distributed, or transmitted in any form or by any means, including photocopying, recording, or other electronic or mechanical methods, without the prior written permission of the publisher, except in the case of brief quotations embodied in critical reviews and certain other noncommercial uses permitted by copyright law.

Let's start this shit!

Arm · **Chest** · **Waist** · **Hips** · **Thigh**

STARTING MEASUREMENTS:

WEIGHT:	
LEFT ARM:	
RIGHT ARM:	
CHEST:	
WAIST:	
HIPS:	
LEFT THIGH:	
RIGHT THIGH:	

SHIT I WANT TO ACHIEVE:

Before Photo

Meals & Shit

	BREAKFAST	LUNCH	DINNER	SNACK
SUNDAY				
MONDAY				
TUESDAY				
WEDNESDAY				
THURSDAY				
FRIDAY				
SATURDAY				

SUNDAY

How I feel today:

Sleep:
Weight:
Protein:
Fat:
Carbs:
Calories:

Water Intake:

Activity:
Time:
Distance:
Sets:
Reps:
Weight Used:
Calories Burned:

MONDAY

How I feel today:

Sleep:
Weight:
Protein:
Fat:
Carbs:
Calories:

Water Intake:

Activity:
Time:
Distance:
Sets:
Reps:
Weight Used:
Calories Burned:

TUESDAY

How I feel today:

Sleep:
Weight:
Protein:
Fat:
Carbs:
Calories:

Water Intake:

Activity:
Time:
Distance:
Sets:
Reps:
Weight Used:
Calories Burned:

WEDNESDAY

How I feel today:

Sleep: _____
Weight: _____
Protein: _____
Fat: _____
Carbs: _____
Calories: _____

Water Intake:

Activity: _____
Time: _____
Distance: _____
Sets: _____
Reps: _____
Weight Used: _____
Calories Burned: _____

THURSDAY

How I feel today:

Sleep: _____
Weight: _____
Protein: _____
Fat: _____
Carbs: _____
Calories: _____

Water Intake:

Activity: _____
Time: _____
Distance: _____
Sets: _____
Reps: _____
Weight Used: _____
Calories Burned: _____

FRIDAY

How I feel today:

Sleep: _____
Weight: _____
Protein: _____
Fat: _____
Carbs: _____
Calories: _____

Water Intake:

Activity: _____
Time: _____
Distance: _____
Sets: _____
Reps: _____
Weight Used: _____
Calories Burned: _____

SATURDAY

How I feel today:

Sleep:
Weight:
Protein:
Fat:
Carbs:
Calories:

Water Intake:

Activity:
Time:
Distance:
Sets:
Reps:
Weight Used:
Calories Burned:

Weekly Progress Tracker

	MEASUREMENT:	LOSS/GAIN:
WEIGHT:		
LEFT ARM:		
RIGHT ARM:		
CHEST:		
WAIST:		
HIPS:		
LEFT THIGH:		
RIGHT THIGH:		

Weekly Goals

Notes

Smash the shit out of your weight loss goals!

Groceries & Shit

Meals & Shit

	BREAKFAST	LUNCH	DINNER	SNACK
SUNDAY				
MONDAY				
TUESDAY				
WEDNESDAY				
THURSDAY				
FRIDAY				
SATURDAY				

SUNDAY

How I feel today:

Sleep: _____
Weight: _____
Protein: _____
Fat: _____
Carbs: _____
Calories: _____

Water Intake:

Activity: _____
Time: _____
Distance: _____
Sets: _____
Reps: _____
Weight Used: _____
Calories Burned: _____

MONDAY

How I feel today:

Sleep: _____
Weight: _____
Protein: _____
Fat: _____
Carbs: _____
Calories: _____

Water Intake:

Activity: _____
Time: _____
Distance: _____
Sets: _____
Reps: _____
Weight Used: _____
Calories Burned: _____

TUESDAY

How I feel today:

Sleep: _____
Weight: _____
Protein: _____
Fat: _____
Carbs: _____
Calories: _____

Water Intake:

Activity: _____
Time: _____
Distance: _____
Sets: _____
Reps: _____
Weight Used: _____
Calories Burned: _____

WEDNESDAY

How I feel today:

Sleep:	
Weight:	
Protein:	
Fat:	
Carbs:	
Calories:	

Water Intake:

Activity:	
Time:	
Distance:	
Sets:	
Reps:	
Weight Used:	
Calories Burned:	

THURSDAY

How I feel today:

Sleep:	
Weight:	
Protein:	
Fat:	
Carbs:	
Calories:	

Water Intake:

Activity:	
Time:	
Distance:	
Sets:	
Reps:	
Weight Used:	
Calories Burned:	

FRIDAY

How I feel today:

Sleep:	
Weight:	
Protein:	
Fat:	
Carbs:	
Calories:	

Water Intake:

Activity:	
Time:	
Distance:	
Sets:	
Reps:	
Weight Used:	
Calories Burned:	

SATURDAY

How I feel today:

Sleep:
Weight:
Protein:
Fat:
Carbs:
Calories:

Water Intake:

Activity:
Time:
Distance:
Sets:
Reps:
Weight Used:
Calories Burned:

Weekly Progress Tracker

MEASUREMENT: LOSS/GAIN:

WEIGHT:

LEFT ARM:

RIGHT ARM:

CHEST:

WAIST:

HIPS:

LEFT THIGH:

RIGHT THIGH:

Weekly Goals

Notes

I won't quit but I will swear the whole time.

Groceries & Shit

Meals & Shit

	BREAKFAST	LUNCH	DINNER	SNACK
SUNDAY				
MONDAY				
TUESDAY				
WEDNESDAY				
THURSDAY				
FRIDAY				
SATURDAY				

SUNDAY

How I feel today:

Sleep:	
Weight:	
Protein:	
Fat:	
Carbs:	
Calories:	

Water Intake:

Activity:	
Time:	
Distance:	
Sets:	
Reps:	
Weight Used:	
Calories Burned:	

MONDAY

How I feel today:

Sleep:	
Weight:	
Protein:	
Fat:	
Carbs:	
Calories:	

Water Intake:

Activity:	
Time:	
Distance:	
Sets:	
Reps:	
Weight Used:	
Calories Burned:	

TUESDAY

How I feel today:

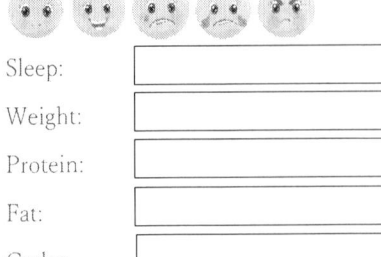

Sleep:	
Weight:	
Protein:	
Fat:	
Carbs:	
Calories:	

Water Intake:

Activity:	
Time:	
Distance:	
Sets:	
Reps:	
Weight Used:	
Calories Burned:	

WEDNESDAY

How I feel today:

Sleep:
Weight:
Protein:
Fat:
Carbs:
Calories:

Water Intake:

Activity:
Time:
Distance:
Sets:
Reps:
Weight Used:
Calories Burned:

THURSDAY

How I feel today:

Sleep:
Weight:
Protein:
Fat:
Carbs:
Calories:

Water Intake:

Activity:
Time:
Distance:
Sets:
Reps:
Weight Used:
Calories Burned:

FRIDAY

How I feel today:

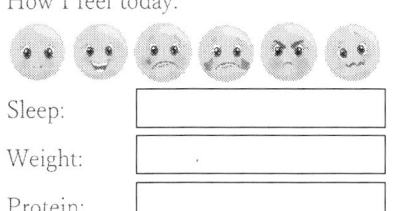

Sleep:
Weight:
Protein:
Fat:
Carbs:
Calories:

Water Intake:

Activity:
Time:
Distance:
Sets:
Reps:
Weight Used:
Calories Burned:

SATURDAY

How I feel today:

Sleep: _____
Weight: _____
Protein: _____
Fat: _____
Carbs: _____
Calories: _____

Water Intake:

Activity: _____
Time: _____
Distance: _____
Sets: _____
Reps: _____
Weight Used: _____
Calories Burned: _____

Weekly Progress Tracker

	MEASUREMENT:	LOSS/GAIN:
WEIGHT:		
LEFT ARM:		
RIGHT ARM:		
CHEST:		
WAIST:		
HIPS:		
LEFT THIGH:		
RIGHT THIGH:		

Weekly Goals

Notes

It's about progress, not fucking being perfect!

Groceries & Shit

Meals & Shit

	BREAKFAST	LUNCH	DINNER	SNACK
SUNDAY				
MONDAY				
TUESDAY				
WEDNESDAY				
THURSDAY				
FRIDAY				
SATURDAY				

SUNDAY

How I feel today:

Sleep:
Weight:
Protein:
Fat:
Carbs:
Calories:

Water Intake:

Activity:
Time:
Distance:
Sets:
Reps:
Weight Used:
Calories Burned:

MONDAY

How I feel today:

Sleep:
Weight:
Protein:
Fat:
Carbs:
Calories:

Water Intake:

Activity:
Time:
Distance:
Sets:
Reps:
Weight Used:
Calories Burned:

TUESDAY

How I feel today:

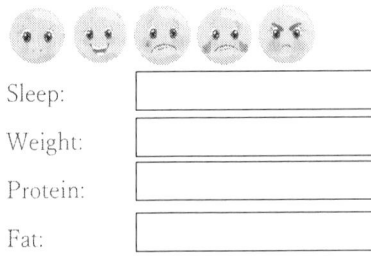

Sleep:
Weight:
Protein:
Fat:
Carbs:
Calories:

Water Intake:

Activity:
Time:
Distance:
Sets:
Reps:
Weight Used:
Calories Burned:

WEDNESDAY

How I feel today:

Sleep:
Weight:
Protein:
Fat:
Carbs:
Calories:

Water Intake:

Activity:
Time:
Distance:
Sets:
Reps:
Weight Used:
Calories Burned:

THURSDAY

How I feel today:

Sleep:
Weight:
Protein:
Fat:
Carbs:
Calories:

Water Intake:

Activity:
Time:
Distance:
Sets:
Reps:
Weight Used:
Calories Burned:

FRIDAY

How I feel today:

Sleep:
Weight:
Protein:
Fat:
Carbs:
Calories:

Water Intake:

Activity:
Time:
Distance:
Sets:
Reps:
Weight Used:
Calories Burned:

SATURDAY

How I feel today:

Sleep:	
Weight:	
Protein:	
Fat:	
Carbs:	
Calories:	

Water Intake:

Activity:	
Time:	
Distance:	
Sets:	
Reps:	
Weight Used:	
Calories Burned:	

Weekly Progress Tracker

	MEASUREMENT:	LOSS/GAIN:
WEIGHT:		
LEFT ARM:		
RIGHT ARM:		
CHEST:		
WAIST:		
HIPS:		
LEFT THIGH:		
RIGHT THIGH:		

Weekly Goals

Notes

You are a badass bitch; you can do this!

Groceries & Shit

Progress Photo

Meals & Shit

	BREAKFAST	LUNCH	DINNER	SNACK
SUNDAY				
MONDAY				
TUESDAY				
WEDNESDAY				
THURSDAY				
FRIDAY				
SATURDAY				

SUNDAY

How I feel today:

Sleep:
Weight:
Protein:
Fat:
Carbs:
Calories:

Water Intake:

Activity:
Time:
Distance:
Sets:
Reps:
Weight Used:
Calories Burned:

MONDAY

How I feel today:

Sleep:
Weight:
Protein:
Fat:
Carbs:
Calories:

Water Intake:

Activity:
Time:
Distance:
Sets:
Reps:
Weight Used:
Calories Burned:

TUESDAY

How I feel today:

Sleep:
Weight:
Protein:
Fat:
Carbs:
Calories:

Water Intake:

Activity:
Time:
Distance:
Sets:
Reps:
Weight Used:
Calories Burned:

WEDNESDAY

How I feel today:

Sleep:
Weight:
Protein:
Fat:
Carbs:
Calories:

Water Intake:

Activity:
Time:
Distance:
Sets:
Reps:
Weight Used:
Calories Burned:

THURSDAY

How I feel today:

Sleep:
Weight:
Protein:
Fat:
Carbs:
Calories:

Water Intake:

Activity:
Time:
Distance:
Sets:
Reps:
Weight Used:
Calories Burned:

FRIDAY

How I feel today:

Sleep:
Weight:
Protein:
Fat:
Carbs:
Calories:

Water Intake:

Activity:
Time:
Distance:
Sets:
Reps:
Weight Used:
Calories Burned:

SATURDAY

How I feel today:

Sleep:
Weight:
Protein:
Fat:
Carbs:
Calories:

Water Intake:

Activity:
Time:
Distance:
Sets:
Reps:
Weight Used:
Calories Burned:

Weekly Progress Tracker

	MEASUREMENT:	LOSS/GAIN:
WEIGHT:		
LEFT ARM:		
RIGHT ARM:		
CHEST:		
WAIST:		
HIPS:		
LEFT THIGH:		
RIGHT THIGH:		

Weekly Goals

Notes

Challenge yourself, get shit done!

Groceries & Shit

Meals & Shit

	BREAKFAST	LUNCH	DINNER	SNACK
SUNDAY				
MONDAY				
TUESDAY				
WEDNESDAY				
THURSDAY				
FRIDAY				
SATURDAY				

SUNDAY

How I feel today:

Sleep:
Weight:
Protein:
Fat:
Carbs:
Calories:

Water Intake:

Activity:
Time:
Distance:
Sets:
Reps:
Weight Used:
Calories Burned:

MONDAY

How I feel today:

Sleep:
Weight:
Protein:
Fat:
Carbs:
Calories:

Water Intake:

Activity:
Time:
Distance:
Sets:
Reps:
Weight Used:
Calories Burned:

TUESDAY

How I feel today:

Sleep:
Weight:
Protein:
Fat:
Carbs:
Calories:

Water Intake:

Activity:
Time:
Distance:
Sets:
Reps:
Weight Used:
Calories Burned:

WEDNESDAY

How I feel today:

Sleep:
Weight:
Protein:
Fat:
Carbs:
Calories:

Water Intake:

Activity:
Time:
Distance:
Sets:
Reps:
Weight Used:
Calories Burned:

THURSDAY

How I feel today:

Sleep:
Weight:
Protein:
Fat:
Carbs:
Calories:

Water Intake:

Activity:
Time:
Distance:
Sets:
Reps:
Weight Used:
Calories Burned:

FRIDAY

How I feel today:

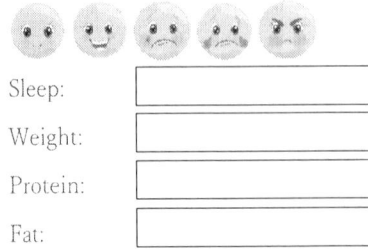

Sleep:
Weight:
Protein:
Fat:
Carbs:
Calories:

Water Intake:

Activity:
Time:
Distance:
Sets:
Reps:
Weight Used:
Calories Burned:

SATURDAY

How I feel today:

Water Intake:

Sleep:

Weight:

Protein:

Fat:

Carbs:

Calories:

Activity:

Time:

Distance:

Sets:

Reps:

Weight Used:

Calories Burned:

Weekly Progress Tracker

	MEASUREMENT:	LOSS/GAIN:
WEIGHT:		
LEFT ARM:		
RIGHT ARM:		
CHEST:		
WAIST:		
HIPS:		
LEFT THIGH:		
RIGHT THIGH:		

Weekly Goals

Notes

Look at you getting healthier and shit!

Groceries & Shit

Meals & Shit

	BREAKFAST	LUNCH	DINNER	SNACK
SUNDAY				
MONDAY				
TUESDAY				
WEDNESDAY				
THURSDAY				
FRIDAY				
SATURDAY				

SUNDAY

How I feel today:

Sleep:
Weight:
Protein:
Fat:
Carbs:
Calories:

Water Intake:

Activity:
Time:
Distance:
Sets:
Reps:
Weight Used:
Calories Burned:

MONDAY

How I feel today:

Sleep:
Weight:
Protein:
Fat:
Carbs:
Calories:

Water Intake:

Activity:
Time:
Distance:
Sets:
Reps:
Weight Used:
Calories Burned:

TUESDAY

How I feel today:

Sleep:
Weight:
Protein:
Fat:
Carbs:
Calories:

Water Intake:

Activity:
Time:
Distance:
Sets:
Reps:
Weight Used:
Calories Burned:

WEDNESDAY

How I feel today:

Sleep:
Weight:
Protein:
Fat:
Carbs:
Calories:

Water Intake:

Activity:
Time:
Distance:
Sets:
Reps:
Weight Used:
Calories Burned:

THURSDAY

How I feel today:

Sleep:
Weight:
Protein:
Fat:
Carbs:
Calories:

Water Intake:

Activity:
Time:
Distance:
Sets:
Reps:
Weight Used:
Calories Burned:

FRIDAY

How I feel today:

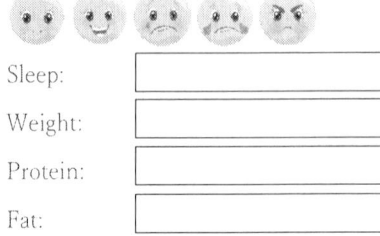

Sleep:
Weight:
Protein:
Fat:
Carbs:
Calories:

Water Intake:

Activity:
Time:
Distance:
Sets:
Reps:
Weight Used:
Calories Burned:

SATURDAY

How I feel today:

Water Intake:

Sleep:	
Weight:	
Protein:	
Fat:	
Carbs:	
Calories:	

Activity:	
Time:	
Distance:	
Sets:	
Reps:	
Weight Used:	
Calories Burned:	

Weekly Progress Tracker

	MEASUREMENT:	LOSS/GAIN:
WEIGHT:		
LEFT ARM:		
RIGHT ARM:		
CHEST:		
WAIST:		
HIPS:		
LEFT THIGH:		
RIGHT THIGH:		

Weekly Goals

Notes

Push past the negativity and bullshit!

Groceries & Shit

Progress Photo

Meals & Shit

	BREAKFAST	LUNCH	DINNER	SNACK
SUNDAY				
MONDAY				
TUESDAY				
WEDNESDAY				
THURSDAY				
FRIDAY				
SATURDAY				

SUNDAY

How I feel today:

Sleep:
Weight:
Protein:
Fat:
Carbs:
Calories:

Water Intake:

Activity:
Time:
Distance:
Sets:
Reps:
Weight Used:
Calories Burned:

MONDAY

How I feel today:

Sleep:
Weight:
Protein:
Fat:
Carbs:
Calories:

Water Intake:

Activity:
Time:
Distance:
Sets:
Reps:
Weight Used:
Calories Burned:

TUESDAY

How I feel today:

Sleep:
Weight:
Protein:
Fat:
Carbs:
Calories:

Water Intake:

Activity:
Time:
Distance:
Sets:
Reps:
Weight Used:
Calories Burned:

WEDNESDAY

How I feel today:

Sleep:
Weight:
Protein:
Fat:
Carbs:
Calories:

Water Intake:

Activity:
Time:
Distance:
Sets:
Reps:
Weight Used:
Calories Burned:

THURSDAY

How I feel today:

Sleep:
Weight:
Protein:
Fat:
Carbs:
Calories:

Water Intake:

Activity:
Time:
Distance:
Sets:
Reps:
Weight Used:
Calories Burned:

FRIDAY

How I feel today:

Sleep:
Weight:
Protein:
Fat:
Carbs:
Calories:

Water Intake:

Activity:
Time:
Distance:
Sets:
Reps:
Weight Used:
Calories Burned:

SATURDAY

How I feel today:

Water Intake:

Sleep:	
Weight:	
Protein:	
Fat:	
Carbs:	
Calories:	

Activity:	
Time:	
Distance:	
Sets:	
Reps:	
Weight Used:	
Calories Burned:	

Weekly Progress Tracker

	MEASUREMENT:	LOSS/GAIN:
WEIGHT:		
LEFT ARM:		
RIGHT ARM:		
CHEST:		
WAIST:		
HIPS:		
LEFT THIGH:		
RIGHT THIGH:		

Weekly Goals

Notes

Celebrate your progress, clap your damn self.

Groceries & Shit

Meals & Shit

	BREAKFAST	LUNCH	DINNER	SNACK
SUNDAY				
MONDAY				
TUESDAY				
WEDNESDAY				
THURSDAY				
FRIDAY				
SATURDAY				

SUNDAY

How I feel today:

Sleep:	
Weight:	
Protein:	
Fat:	
Carbs:	
Calories:	

Water Intake:

Activity:	
Time:	
Distance:	
Sets:	
Reps:	
Weight Used:	
Calories Burned:	

MONDAY

How I feel today:

Sleep:	
Weight:	
Protein:	
Fat:	
Carbs:	
Calories:	

Water Intake:

Activity:	
Time:	
Distance:	
Sets:	
Reps:	
Weight Used:	
Calories Burned:	

TUESDAY

How I feel today:

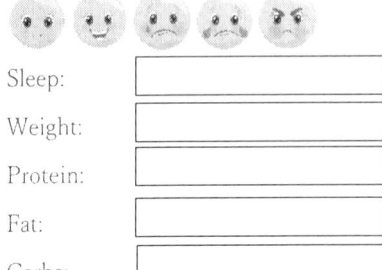

Sleep:	
Weight:	
Protein:	
Fat:	
Carbs:	
Calories:	

Water Intake:

Activity:	
Time:	
Distance:	
Sets:	
Reps:	
Weight Used:	
Calories Burned:	

WEDNESDAY

How I feel today:

Sleep:
Weight:
Protein:
Fat:
Carbs:
Calories:

Water Intake:

Activity:
Time:
Distance:
Sets:
Reps:
Weight Used:
Calories Burned:

THURSDAY

How I feel today:

Sleep:
Weight:
Protein:
Fat:
Carbs:
Calories:

Water Intake:

Activity:
Time:
Distance:
Sets:
Reps:
Weight Used:
Calories Burned:

FRIDAY

How I feel today:

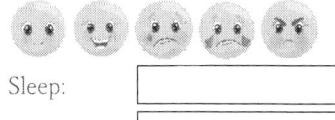

Sleep:
Weight:
Protein:
Fat:
Carbs:
Calories:

Water Intake:

Activity:
Time:
Distance:
Sets:
Reps:
Weight Used:
Calories Burned:

SATURDAY

How I feel today:

Sleep:	
Weight:	
Protein:	
Fat:	
Carbs:	
Calories:	

Water Intake:

Activity:	
Time:	
Distance:	
Sets:	
Reps:	
Weight Used:	
Calories Burned:	

Weekly Progress Tracker

	MEASUREMENT:	LOSS/GAIN:
WEIGHT:		
LEFT ARM:		
RIGHT ARM:		
CHEST:		
WAIST:		
HIPS:		
LEFT THIGH:		
RIGHT THIGH:		

Weekly Goals

Notes

Getting fit AF!

Groceries & Shit

Meals & Shit

	BREAKFAST	LUNCH	DINNER	SNACK
SUNDAY				
MONDAY				
TUESDAY				
WEDNESDAY				
THURSDAY				
FRIDAY				
SATURDAY				

SUNDAY

How I feel today:

Sleep:
Weight:
Protein:
Fat:
Carbs:
Calories:

Water Intake:

Activity:
Time:
Distance:
Sets:
Reps:
Weight Used:
Calories Burned:

MONDAY

How I feel today:

Sleep:
Weight:
Protein:
Fat:
Carbs:
Calories:

Water Intake:

Activity:
Time:
Distance:
Sets:
Reps:
Weight Used:
Calories Burned:

TUESDAY

How I feel today:

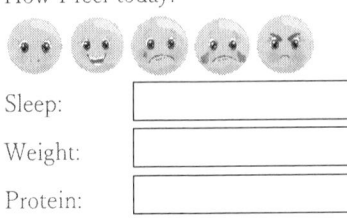

Sleep:
Weight:
Protein:
Fat:
Carbs:
Calories:

Water Intake:

Activity:
Time:
Distance:
Sets:
Reps:
Weight Used:
Calories Burned:

WEDNESDAY

How I feel today:

Sleep:
Weight:
Protein:
Fat:
Carbs:
Calories:

Water Intake:

Activity:
Time:
Distance:
Sets:
Reps:
Weight Used:
Calories Burned:

THURSDAY

How I feel today:

Sleep:
Weight:
Protein:
Fat:
Carbs:
Calories:

Water Intake:

Activity:
Time:
Distance:
Sets:
Reps:
Weight Used:
Calories Burned:

FRIDAY

How I feel today:

Sleep:
Weight:
Protein:
Fat:
Carbs:
Calories:

Water Intake:

Activity:
Time:
Distance:
Sets:
Reps:
Weight Used:
Calories Burned:

SATURDAY

How I feel today:

Water Intake:

Sleep:		Activity:	
Weight:		Time:	
Protein:		Distance:	
Fat:		Sets:	
Carbs:		Reps:	
Calories:		Weight Used:	
		Calories Burned:	

Weekly Progress Tracker

	MEASUREMENT:	LOSS/GAIN:
WEIGHT:		
LEFT ARM:		
RIGHT ARM:		
CHEST:		
WAIST:		
HIPS:		
LEFT THIGH:		
RIGHT THIGH:		

Weekly Goals

Notes

Fuck the doubt!

Groceries & Shit

Meals & Shit

	BREAKFAST	LUNCH	DINNER	SNACK
SUNDAY				
MONDAY				
TUESDAY				
WEDNESDAY				
THURSDAY				
FRIDAY				
SATURDAY				

SUNDAY

How I feel today:

Sleep:
Weight:
Protein:
Fat:
Carbs:
Calories:

Water Intake:

Activity:
Time:
Distance:
Sets:
Reps:
Weight Used:
Calories Burned:

MONDAY

How I feel today:

Sleep:
Weight:
Protein:
Fat:
Carbs:
Calories:

Water Intake:

Activity:
Time:
Distance:
Sets:
Reps:
Weight Used:
Calories Burned:

TUESDAY

How I feel today:

Sleep:
Weight:
Protein:
Fat:
Carbs:
Calories:

Water Intake:

Activity:
Time:
Distance:
Sets:
Reps:
Weight Used:
Calories Burned:

WEDNESDAY

How I feel today:

Sleep: _____
Weight: _____
Protein: _____
Fat: _____
Carbs: _____
Calories: _____

Water Intake:

Activity: _____
Time: _____
Distance: _____
Sets: _____
Reps: _____
Weight Used: _____
Calories Burned: _____

THURSDAY

How I feel today:

Sleep: _____
Weight: _____
Protein: _____
Fat: _____
Carbs: _____
Calories: _____

Water Intake:

Activity: _____
Time: _____
Distance: _____
Sets: _____
Reps: _____
Weight Used: _____
Calories Burned: _____

FRIDAY

How I feel today:

Sleep: _____
Weight: _____
Protein: _____
Fat: _____
Carbs: _____
Calories: _____

Water Intake:

Activity: _____
Time: _____
Distance: _____
Sets: _____
Reps: _____
Weight Used: _____
Calories Burned: _____

SATURDAY

How I feel today:

Water Intake:

Sleep:		Activity:	
Weight:		Time:	
Protein:		Distance:	
Fat:		Sets:	
Carbs:		Reps:	
Calories:		Weight Used:	
		Calories Burned:	

Weekly Progress Tracker

	MEASUREMENT:	LOSS/GAIN:
WEIGHT:		
LEFT ARM:		
RIGHT ARM:		
CHEST:		
WAIST:		
HIPS:		
LEFT THIGH:		
RIGHT THIGH:		

Weekly Goals

Notes

Get up and kick ass today!

Groceries & Shit

Progress Photo

Meals & Shit

	BREAKFAST	LUNCH	DINNER	SNACK
SUNDAY				
MONDAY				
TUESDAY				
WEDNESDAY				
THURSDAY				
FRIDAY				
SATURDAY				

SUNDAY

How I feel today:

Sleep:
Weight:
Protein:
Fat:
Carbs:
Calories:

Water Intake:

Activity:
Time:
Distance:
Sets:
Reps:
Weight Used:
Calories Burned:

MONDAY

How I feel today:

Sleep:
Weight:
Protein:
Fat:
Carbs:
Calories:

Water Intake:

Activity:
Time:
Distance:
Sets:
Reps:
Weight Used:
Calories Burned:

TUESDAY

How I feel today:

Sleep:
Weight:
Protein:
Fat:
Carbs:
Calories:

Water Intake:

Activity:
Time:
Distance:
Sets:
Reps:
Weight Used:
Calories Burned:

WEDNESDAY

How I feel today:

Sleep: _____
Weight: _____
Protein: _____
Fat: _____
Carbs: _____
Calories: _____

Water Intake:

Activity: _____
Time: _____
Distance: _____
Sets: _____
Reps: _____
Weight Used: _____
Calories Burned: _____

THURSDAY

How I feel today:

Sleep: _____
Weight: _____
Protein: _____
Fat: _____
Carbs: _____
Calories: _____

Water Intake:

Activity: _____
Time: _____
Distance: _____
Sets: _____
Reps: _____
Weight Used: _____
Calories Burned: _____

FRIDAY

How I feel today:

Sleep: _____
Weight: _____
Protein: _____
Fat: _____
Carbs: _____
Calories: _____

Water Intake:

Activity: _____
Time: _____
Distance: _____
Sets: _____
Reps: _____
Weight Used: _____
Calories Burned: _____

SATURDAY

How I feel today:

Sleep:		Water Intake:	
Weight:		Activity:	
Protein:		Time:	
Fat:		Distance:	
Carbs:		Sets:	
Calories:		Reps:	
		Weight Used:	
		Calories Burned:	

Weekly Progress Tracker

	MEASUREMENT:	LOSS/GAIN:
WEIGHT:		
LEFT ARM:		
RIGHT ARM:		
CHEST:		
WAIST:		
HIPS:		
LEFT THIGH:		
RIGHT THIGH:		

Weekly Goals

Notes

Never forget, you're fucking awesome!

Groceries & Shit

Meals & Shit

	BREAKFAST	LUNCH	DINNER	SNACK
SUNDAY				
MONDAY				
TUESDAY				
WEDNESDAY				
THURSDAY				
FRIDAY				
SATURDAY				

SUNDAY

How I feel today:

Sleep:
Weight:
Protein:
Fat:
Carbs:
Calories:

Water Intake:

Activity:
Time:
Distance:
Sets:
Reps:
Weight Used:
Calories Burned:

MONDAY

How I feel today:

Sleep:
Weight:
Protein:
Fat:
Carbs:
Calories:

Water Intake:

Activity:
Time:
Distance:
Sets:
Reps:
Weight Used:
Calories Burned:

TUESDAY

How I feel today:

Sleep:
Weight:
Protein:
Fat:
Carbs:
Calories:

Water Intake:

Activity:
Time:
Distance:
Sets:
Reps:
Weight Used:
Calories Burned:

WEDNESDAY

How I feel today:

Sleep: _____
Weight: _____
Protein: _____
Fat: _____
Carbs: _____
Calories: _____

Water Intake:

Activity: _____
Time: _____
Distance: _____
Sets: _____
Reps: _____
Weight Used: _____
Calories Burned: _____

THURSDAY

How I feel today:

Sleep: _____
Weight: _____
Protein: _____
Fat: _____
Carbs: _____
Calories: _____

Water Intake:

Activity: _____
Time: _____
Distance: _____
Sets: _____
Reps: _____
Weight Used: _____
Calories Burned: _____

FRIDAY

How I feel today:

Sleep: _____
Weight: _____
Protein: _____
Fat: _____
Carbs: _____
Calories: _____

Water Intake:

Activity: _____
Time: _____
Distance: _____
Sets: _____
Reps: _____
Weight Used: _____
Calories Burned: _____

SATURDAY

How I feel today:

Sleep: _____
Weight: _____
Protein: _____
Fat: _____
Carbs: _____
Calories: _____

Water Intake:

Activity: _____
Time: _____
Distance: _____
Sets: _____
Reps: _____
Weight Used: _____
Calories Burned: _____

Weekly Progress Tracker

	MEASUREMENT:	LOSS/GAIN:
WEIGHT:		
LEFT ARM:		
RIGHT ARM:		
CHEST:		
WAIST:		
HIPS:		
LEFT THIGH:		
RIGHT THIGH:		

Weekly Goals

Notes

Be fucking kind to yourself.

Groceries & Shit

Meals & Shit

	BREAKFAST	LUNCH	DINNER	SNACK
SUNDAY				
MONDAY				
TUESDAY				
WEDNESDAY				
THURSDAY				
FRIDAY				
SATURDAY				

SUNDAY

How I feel today:

Sleep:
Weight:
Protein:
Fat:
Carbs:
Calories:

Water Intake:

Activity:
Time:
Distance:
Sets:
Reps:
Weight Used:
Calories Burned:

MONDAY

How I feel today:

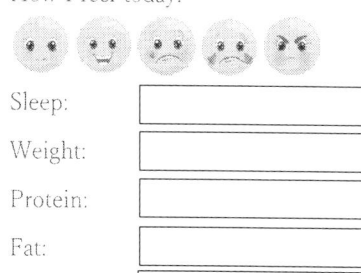

Sleep:
Weight:
Protein:
Fat:
Carbs:
Calories:

Water Intake:

Activity:
Time:
Distance:
Sets:
Reps:
Weight Used:
Calories Burned:

TUESDAY

How I feel today:

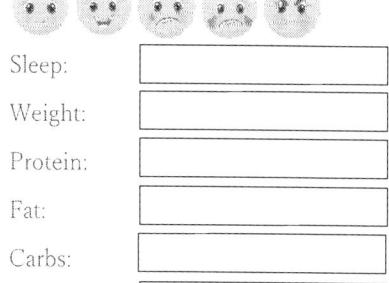

Sleep:
Weight:
Protein:
Fat:
Carbs:
Calories:

Water Intake:

Activity:
Time:
Distance:
Sets:
Reps:
Weight Used:
Calories Burned:

WEDNESDAY

How I feel today:

Sleep:
Weight:
Protein:
Fat:
Carbs:
Calories:

Water Intake:

Activity:
Time:
Distance:
Sets:
Reps:
Weight Used:
Calories Burned:

THURSDAY

How I feel today:

Sleep:
Weight:
Protein:
Fat:
Carbs:
Calories:

Water Intake:

Activity:
Time:
Distance:
Sets:
Reps:
Weight Used:
Calories Burned:

FRIDAY

How I feel today:

Sleep:
Weight:
Protein:
Fat:
Carbs:
Calories:

Water Intake:

Activity:
Time:
Distance:
Sets:
Reps:
Weight Used:
Calories Burned:

SATURDAY

How I feel today:

Water Intake:

Sleep:		Activity:	
Weight:		Time:	
Protein:		Distance:	
Fat:		Sets:	
Carbs:		Reps:	
Calories:		Weight Used:	
		Calories Burned:	

Weekly Progress Tracker

	MEASUREMENT:	LOSS/GAIN:
WEIGHT:		
LEFT ARM:		
RIGHT ARM:		
CHEST:		
WAIST:		
HIPS:		
LEFT THIGH:		
RIGHT THIGH:		

Weekly Goals

Notes

Be a badass with a good ass!

Groceries & Shit

Progress Photo

Meals & Shit

	BREAKFAST	LUNCH	DINNER	SNACK
SUNDAY				
MONDAY				
TUESDAY				
WEDNESDAY				
THURSDAY				
FRIDAY				
SATURDAY				

SUNDAY

How I feel today:

Sleep:
Weight:
Protein:
Fat:
Carbs:
Calories:

Water Intake:

Activity:
Time:
Distance:
Sets:
Reps:
Weight Used:
Calories Burned:

MONDAY

How I feel today:

Sleep:
Weight:
Protein:
Fat:
Carbs:
Calories:

Water Intake:

Activity:
Time:
Distance:
Sets:
Reps:
Weight Used:
Calories Burned:

TUESDAY

How I feel today:

Sleep:
Weight:
Protein:
Fat:
Carbs:
Calories:

Water Intake:

Activity:
Time:
Distance:
Sets:
Reps:
Weight Used:
Calories Burned:

WEDNESDAY

How I feel today:

Sleep:
Weight:
Protein:
Fat:
Carbs:
Calories:

Water Intake:

Activity:
Time:
Distance:
Sets:
Reps:
Weight Used:
Calories Burned:

THURSDAY

How I feel today:

Sleep:
Weight:
Protein:
Fat:
Carbs:
Calories:

Water Intake:

Activity:
Time:
Distance:
Sets:
Reps:
Weight Used:
Calories Burned:

FRIDAY

How I feel today:

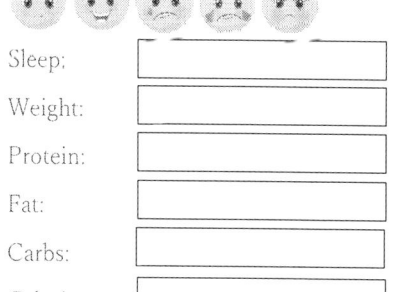

Sleep:
Weight:
Protein:
Fat:
Carbs:
Calories:

Water Intake:

Activity:
Time:
Distance:
Sets:
Reps:
Weight Used:
Calories Burned:

SATURDAY

How I feel today:

Sleep:

Weight:

Protein:

Fat:

Carbs:

Calories:

Water Intake:

Activity:

Time:

Distance:

Sets:

Reps:

Weight Used:

Calories Burned:

Weekly Progress Tracker

	MEASUREMENT:	LOSS/GAIN:
WEIGHT:		
LEFT ARM:		
RIGHT ARM:		
CHEST:		
WAIST:		
HIPS:		
LEFT THIGH:		
RIGHT THIGH:		

Weekly Goals

Notes

Go harder, do the shit you think you can't do

Groceries & Shit

Meals & Shit

	BREAKFAST	LUNCH	DINNER	SNACK
SUNDAY				
MONDAY				
TUESDAY				
WEDNESDAY				
THURSDAY				
FRIDAY				
SATURDAY				

SUNDAY

How I feel today:

Sleep:
Weight:
Protein:
Fat:
Carbs:
Calories:

Water Intake:

Activity:
Time:
Distance:
Sets:
Reps:
Weight Used:
Calories Burned:

MONDAY

How I feel today:

Sleep:
Weight:
Protein:
Fat:
Carbs:
Calories:

Water Intake:

Activity:
Time:
Distance:
Sets:
Reps:
Weight Used:
Calories Burned:

TUESDAY

How I feel today:

Sleep:
Weight:
Protein:
Fat:
Carbs:
Calories:

Water Intake:

Activity:
Time:
Distance:
Sets:
Reps:
Weight Used:
Calories Burned:

WEDNESDAY

How I feel today:

Sleep:
Weight:
Protein:
Fat:
Carbs:
Calories:

Water Intake:

Activity:
Time:
Distance:
Sets:
Reps:
Weight Used:
Calories Burned:

THURSDAY

How I feel today:

Sleep:
Weight:
Protein:
Fat:
Carbs:
Calories:

Water Intake:

Activity:
Time:
Distance:
Sets:
Reps:
Weight Used:
Calories Burned:

FRIDAY

How I feel today:

Sleep:
Weight:
Protein:
Fat:
Carbs:
Calories:

Water Intake:

Activity:
Time:
Distance:
Sets:
Reps:
Weight Used:
Calories Burned:

SATURDAY

How I feel today:

Sleep:	
Weight:	
Protein:	
Fat:	
Carbs:	
Calories:	

Water Intake:

Activity:	
Time:	
Distance:	
Sets:	
Reps:	
Weight Used:	
Calories Burned:	

Weekly Progress Tracker

	MEASUREMENT:	LOSS/GAIN:
WEIGHT:		
LEFT ARM:		
RIGHT ARM:		
CHEST:		
WAIST:		
HIPS:		
LEFT THIGH:		
RIGHT THIGH:		

Weekly Goals

You're getting close as fuck to your goals!

Groceries & Shit

Meals & Shit

	BREAKFAST	LUNCH	DINNER	SNACK
SUNDAY				
MONDAY				
TUESDAY				
WEDNESDAY				
THURSDAY				
FRIDAY				
SATURDAY				

SUNDAY

How I feel today:

Sleep:	
Weight:	
Protein:	
Fat:	
Carbs:	
Calories:	

Water Intake:

Activity:	
Time:	
Distance:	
Sets:	
Reps:	
Weight Used:	
Calories Burned:	

MONDAY

How I feel today:

Sleep:	
Weight:	
Protein:	
Fat:	
Carbs:	
Calories:	

Water Intake:

Activity:	
Time:	
Distance:	
Sets:	
Reps:	
Weight Used:	
Calories Burned:	

TUESDAY

How I feel today:

Sleep:	
Weight:	
Protein:	
Fat:	
Carbs:	
Calories:	

Water Intake:

Activity:	
Time:	
Distance:	
Sets:	
Reps:	
Weight Used:	
Calories Burned:	

WEDNESDAY

How I feel today:

Sleep: _____
Weight: _____
Protein: _____
Fat: _____
Carbs: _____
Calories: _____

Water Intake:

Activity: _____
Time: _____
Distance: _____
Sets: _____
Reps: _____
Weight Used: _____
Calories Burned: _____

THURSDAY

How I feel today:

Sleep: _____
Weight: _____
Protein: _____
Fat: _____
Carbs: _____
Calories: _____

Water Intake:

Activity: _____
Time: _____
Distance: _____
Sets: _____
Reps: _____
Weight Used: _____
Calories Burned: _____

FRIDAY

How I feel today:

Sleep: _____
Weight: _____
Protein: _____
Fat: _____
Carbs: _____
Calories: _____

Water Intake:

Activity: _____
Time: _____
Distance: _____
Sets: _____
Reps: _____
Weight Used: _____
Calories Burned: _____

SATURDAY

How I feel today:

Water Intake:

Sleep:

Weight:

Protein:

Fat:

Carbs:

Calories:

Activity:

Time:

Distance:

Sets:

Reps:

Weight Used:

Calories Burned:

Weekly Progress Tracker

	MEASUREMENT:	LOSS/GAIN:
WEIGHT:		
LEFT ARM:		
RIGHT ARM:		
CHEST:		
WAIST:		
HIPS:		
LEFT THIGH:		
RIGHT THIGH:		

Weekly Goals

Notes

Shit is hard but you'll soon get the reward!

Groceries & Shit

Meals & Shit

	BREAKFAST	LUNCH	DINNER	SNACK
SUNDAY				
MONDAY				
TUESDAY				
WEDNESDAY				
THURSDAY				
FRIDAY				
SATURDAY				

SUNDAY

How I feel today:

Sleep:	
Weight:	
Protein:	
Fat:	
Carbs:	
Calories:	

Water Intake:

Activity:	
Time:	
Distance:	
Sets:	
Reps:	
Weight Used:	
Calories Burned:	

MONDAY

How I feel today:

Sleep:	
Weight:	
Protein:	
Fat:	
Carbs:	
Calories:	

Water Intake:

Activity:	
Time:	
Distance:	
Sets:	
Reps:	
Weight Used:	
Calories Burned:	

TUESDAY

How I feel today:

Sleep:	
Weight:	
Protein:	
Fat:	
Carbs:	
Calories:	

Water Intake:

Activity:	
Time:	
Distance:	
Sets:	
Reps:	
Weight Used:	
Calories Burned:	

WEDNESDAY

How I feel today:

Sleep:
Weight:
Protein:
Fat:
Carbs:
Calories:

Water Intake:

Activity:
Time:
Distance:
Sets:
Reps:
Weight Used:
Calories Burned:

THURSDAY

How I feel today:

Sleep:
Weight:
Protein:
Fat:
Carbs:
Calories:

Water Intake:

Activity:
Time:
Distance:
Sets:
Reps:
Weight Used:
Calories Burned:

FRIDAY

How I feel today:

Sleep:
Weight:
Protein:
Fat:
Carbs:
Calories:

Water Intake:

Activity:
Time:
Distance:
Sets:
Reps:
Weight Used:
Calories Burned:

SATURDAY

How I feel today:

Sleep:

Weight:

Protein:

Fat:

Carbs:

Calories:

Water Intake:

Activity:

Time:

Distance:

Sets:

Reps:

Weight Used:

Calories Burned:

Weekly Progress Tracker

	MEASUREMENT:	LOSS/GAIN:
WEIGHT:		
LEFT ARM:		
RIGHT ARM:		
CHEST:		
WAIST:		
HIPS:		
LEFT THIGH:		
RIGHT THIGH:		

Weekly Goals

You fucking did it!

Groceries & Shit

After Photo

Made in the USA
Coppell, TX
25 September 2022